Contents

Features to help you succeed ... 4

A1 Working within the health and science sector ... 5

A2 The healthcare sector ... 10

A3 Health, safety and environmental regulations in the health and science sector ... 17

A4 Health and safety regulations applicable in the healthcare sector ... 22

A5 Managing information and data within the health and science sector ... 25

A6 Managing personal information ... 32

A7 Good scientific and clinical practice ... 38

A8 Providing person-centred care ... 42

A9 Health and wellbeing ... 50

A10 Infection prevention and control in health specific settings ... 57

A11 Safeguarding ... 62

B1 Core science concepts ... 69

B2 Further science concepts in health ... 76

Answers can be found online at www.hachettelearning.com/answers-and-extras

Health T Level Exam Practice Workbook

Features to help you succeed

Recall activities
Each topic area starts with **recall activities** that will help you to remember important information you will need when answering exam questions. These activities include mind maps, matching exercises and filling in missing words in tables, sentences or diagrams.

Hint/Tip
Some short-answer and longer-answer questions include **Hints** or **Tips** next to them to give you extra advice on how to approach the question. **Hints** may suggest key points to consider when answering the question, while **Tips** explain how to answer the question, what important words included in the question mean or give guidance on common mistakes students make when answering these types of questions.

Write your answer
All questions will have spaces for you to write your answers.

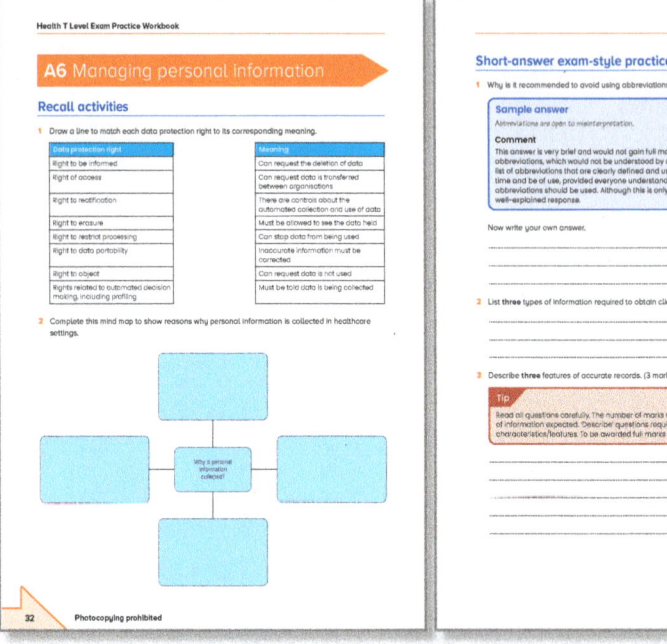

Sample answers
Sample student answers are provided for some questions. These will help you understand how to gain the most marks and may ask you to think about the strengths and weaknesses of the answer and how it could be improved.

Plan your answer
Some questions will also include guidance and space to support you to **plan your answer** before you answer the question. They may identify and explain key words for you, provide tables for you to complete to help you to plan and structure your answer, or include partially completed answers.

Short-answer exam practice
Short-answer exam practice questions help you to practise answering multiple-choice and short-answer exam questions that are typically worth 1–4 marks.

Longer-answer exam practice
Longer-answer exam practice questions will help you to practise answering extended response questions typically worth 5–12 marks. These questions will usually include a context or scenario.

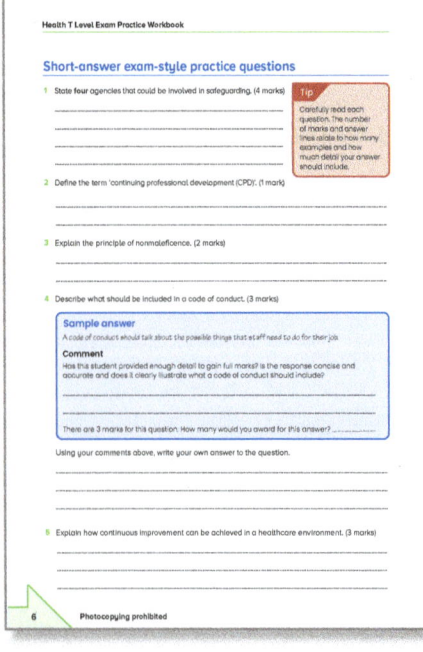
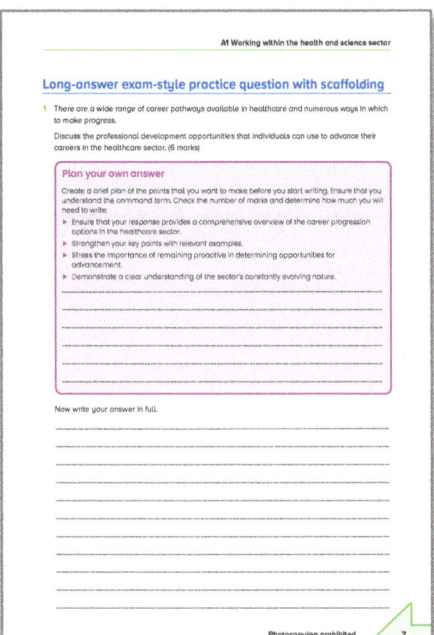

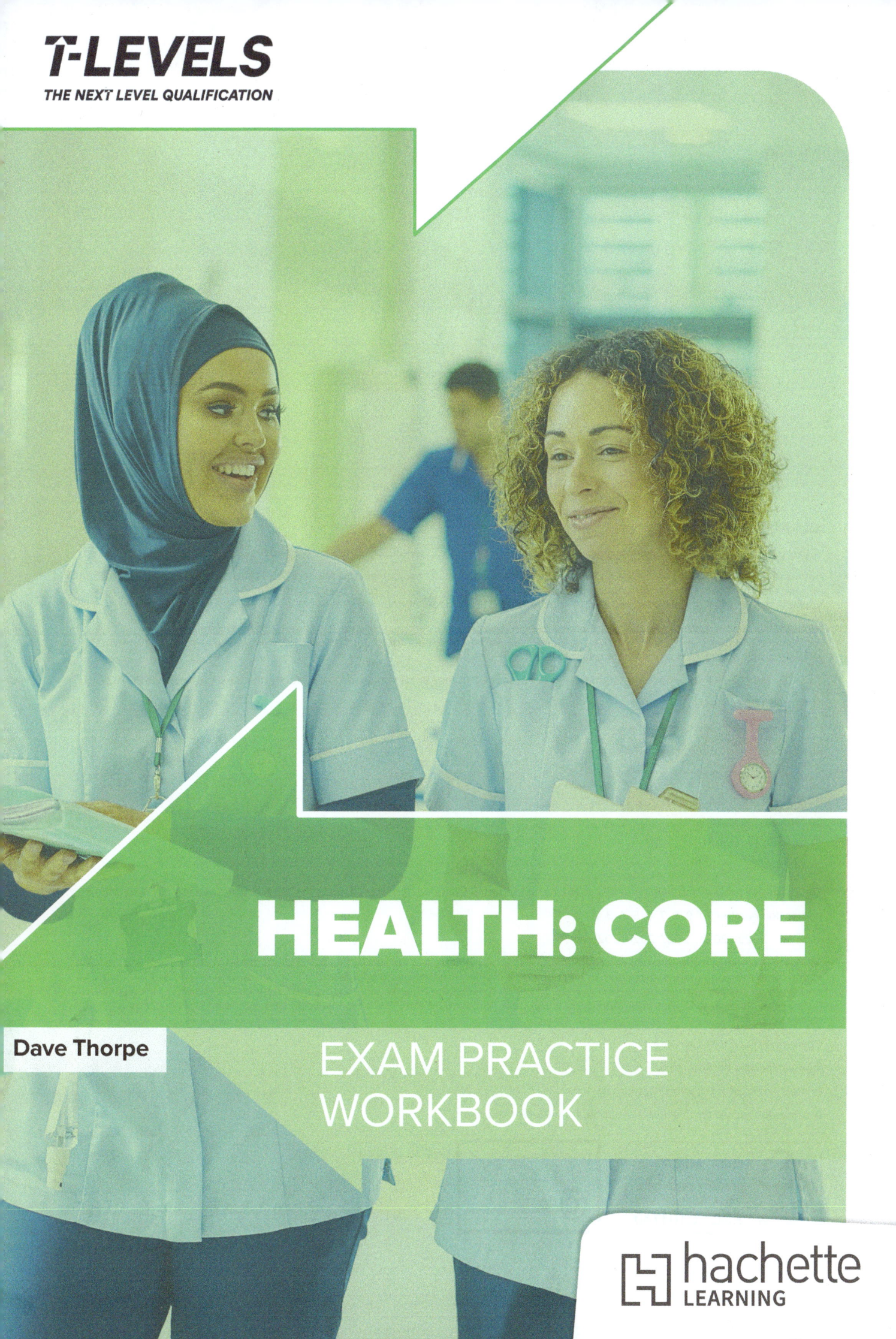

Acknowledgements

With thanks to Judith Adams for reviewing the manuscript for Health T Level Exam Practice Workbook.

Although every effort has been made to ensure that website addresses are correct at time of going to press, Hachette Learning cannot be held responsible for the content of any website mentioned in this book. It is sometimes possible to find a relocated web page by typing in the address of the home page for a website in the URL window of your browser.

Hachette UK's policy is to use papers that are natural, renewable and recyclable products and made from wood grown in well-managed forests and other controlled sources. The logging and manufacturing processes are expected to conform to the environmental regulations of the country of origin.

To order, please visit www.hachettelearning.com or contact Customer Service at education@hachette.co.uk / +44 (0)1235 827827.

ISBN: 978 1 0360 0698 3

© Hodder & Stoughton Limited 2025

First published in 2025 by Hachette Learning,

An Hachette UK Company

Carmelite House

50 Victoria Embankment

London EC4Y 0DZ

www.hachettelearning.com

The authorised representative in the EEA is Hachette Ireland, 8 Castlecourt Centre, Dublin 15, D15 XTP3, Ireland (email: info@hbgi.ie)

Impression number 10 9 8 7 6 5 4 3 2

Year   2029 2028 2027 2026 2025

All rights reserved. Apart from any use permitted under UK copyright law, no part of this publication may be reproduced or transmitted in any form or by any means, electronic or mechanical, including photocopying and recording, or held within any information storage and retrieval system, without permission in writing from the publisher or under licence from the Copyright Licensing Agency Limited. Further details of such licences (for reprographic reproduction) may be obtained from the Copyright Licensing Agency Limited, www.cla.co.uk

Cover photo © iStock.com/sturti

Typeset in India by Aptara Inc.

Printed in the UK BY Ashford Colour Ltd

A catalogue record for this title is available from the British Library.

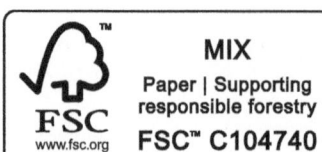
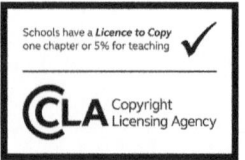

A1 Working within the health and science sector

Recall activities

1   Complete the table to explain the purpose of each key policy.

Policy	Purpose
Equality, diversity and inclusion policy	
Safeguarding policy	
Disciplinary policy	
Grievance policy	

2   Fill in the gaps to complete the definitions. Use the list of words below.

specific	payment	competent	independently
university	reasonable	equal	short
staff	summer	opportunity	everybody

a   **Inclusion**: Ensuring that .... has a voice and a means to participate, which may involve making .... adjustments to usual processes, to be included as an .... to others.

b   **Scholarship**: An .... available for students studying .... subjects at a university. It is a grant or .... of fees, which may be part or full payment.

c   **Autonomy**: Healthcare .... must respect the .... decisions made by an individual as they have the right to make them ....

d   **Internship**: Usually relatively .... and often taking place during the .... months, as many are designed for .... students.

Short-answer exam-style practice questions

1 State **four** agencies that could be involved in safeguarding. (4 marks)

....

....

....

....

> **Tip**
>
> Carefully read each question. The number of marks and answer lines relate to how many examples and how much detail your answer should include.

2 Define the term 'continuing professional development (CPD)'. (1 mark)

....

....

3 Explain the principle of nonmaleficence. (2 marks)

....

....

4 Describe what should be included in a code of conduct. (3 marks)

> **Sample answer**
>
> *A code of conduct should talk about the possible things that staff need to do for their job.*
>
> **Comment**
>
> Has this student provided enough detail to gain full marks? Is the response concise and accurate, and does it clearly illustrate what a code of conduct should include?
>
> ....
>
> ....
>
> There are 3 marks for this question. How many would you award for this answer? ....

Using your comments above, write your own answer to the question.

....

....

....

5 Explain how continuous improvement can be achieved in a healthcare environment. (3 marks)

....

....

....

A1 Working within the health and science sector

Long-answer exam-style practice question with scaffolding

1 There is a wide range of career pathways available in healthcare and numerous ways in which to make progress.

   Discuss the professional development opportunities that individuals can use to advance their careers in the healthcare sector. (6 marks)

> **Plan your own answer**
>
> Create a brief plan of the points that you want to make before you start writing. Ensure that you understand the command term. Check the number of marks and determine how much you will need to write:
> - Ensure that your response provides a comprehensive overview of the career progression options in the healthcare sector.
> - Strengthen your key points with relevant examples.
> - Stress the importance of remaining proactive in determining opportunities for advancement.
> - Demonstrate a clear understanding of the sector's constantly evolving nature.
>
> ....
> ....
> ....
> ....
> ....

Now write your answer in full.

....
....
....
....
....
....
....
....
....
....

Long-answer exam-style practice questions

1 Charlie is 79 years old and has dementia. This means that he can become confused easily and has poor short-term memory. Charlie's independence has been restricted and he lacks the capacity to make important decisions. Explain the principle of autonomy and how informed consent would impact on the decision-making process for Charlie. (9 marks, plus 3 marks for quality of written communication (QWC))

Hint

Consider the impact of loss of capacity and autonomy. When lucid, how might this make Charlie feel? Losing the ability to make important choices for yourself can be distressing and may prompt negative responses and behaviour. How would informed consent be obtained and who might need to be involved in this process?

A1 Working within the health and science sector

2 Amir would like to become a nurse. He gained seven GCSEs at grade 5 or above but has not yet taken any further qualifications. Outline the potential nursing qualifications that might be open to him now and the career progression options open to him once he gains those qualifications.
(9 marks, plus 3 marks for QWC)

> **Hint**
> Make sure your answer covers both the qualifications that Amir would be able to undertake now and describes potential ways he could then progress further. Keep your answer focused on the career path described in the question.

A2 The healthcare sector

Recall activities

1 Construct a mind map that illustrates the **five** potential barriers to accessing services. Include one relevant example for each.

2 Draw a line between the type of care and the corresponding example of that type of care.

Term
Primary Care
Secondary Care
Tertiary Care

Example
Inpatients/outpatients
Long-term care, hospice, highly specialised care
GP, A&E, dentist, school nurse

3 In 1945, the three essential principles that the NHS should be based on were developed. Fill in the gaps to complete these three statements.

   a ………………………………………………………… should be entitled to use it.

   b Healthcare provided should be …………………………………………………………
      of …………………………………………………………

   c It should be based on ………………………………………………………… rather than the ability to pay for it.

4 Identify the main features of primary care. Try to include as many as possible.

1	
2	
3	
4	
5	
6	

Short-answer exam-style questions

1 Outline **four** reasons why health and social care practitioners should adhere to their organisation's policies. (4 marks)

....

....

....

....

....

....

2 Define the term 'evidence-based practice'. (2 marks)

....

....

3 Jamal is part of a multi-disciplinary team caring for a patient who has dementia. State **three** examples of different individuals or agencies that would also be a part of this multi-disciplinary team. (3 marks)

....

....

....

4 Describe **four** benefits of public health provision. (4 marks)

....

....

....

....

....

....

> **Tip**
>
> Look at the number of marks next to each question. Question 4 requires four distinct benefits to gain full marks. Write in sentences and ensure your response is concise and relevant to the question.

5 Describe how multidisciplinary teams work together effectively. (4 marks)

> **Sample answer**
>
> Multidisciplinary teams work together. They should include specific roles. It is important they share relevant information.
>
> **Comment**
>
> Does this sample answer the question sufficiently or would it benefit from being described in a little more detail? Would you change or add anything to improve clarity? What else could be added? How many marks out of 4 does this answer deserve? What could you improve to gain full marks?
>
> ....
>
> ....
>
> ....
>
> ....

Now construct your own response.

....
....
....
....
....
....

Long-answer exam-style practice questions with scaffolding

1 A busy GP surgery's waiting times have doubled in the last three years and many appointments are being taken up by patients who could be effectively managed through pharmacy or online advice. The surgery is considering whether to introduce AI to help tackle the issue.

Analyse the potential impact of AI on waiting times, including challenges and opportunities. (9 marks, plus 3 marks for QWC).

> **Sample answer**
> Future developments in the healthcare sector have the potential to significantly impact care provision, presenting both challenges and opportunities. Some of these developments include advancements in technology, changes in healthcare policy and regulation, shifts in demographics and patient needs, and the evolving role of healthcare professionals.
>
> **Comment**
> This is an extract from an answer for this 9-mark question. Does it provide enough relevant information? Does it answer the question or just provide an introduction? Consider what you could change or add to develop the response.
>
> ....
> ....
> ....
> ....
> ....
> ....

Write **two** additional paragraphs, each with a different focus, for example, AI and one other to develop your answer.

....
....
....

Health T Level Exam Practice Workbook

....
....
....
....
....
....
....
....
....
....
....
....

2 Describe the possible impact of the COVID-19 pandemic on vulnerable individuals living in a care home setting. (6 marks)

> **Plan your own answer**
>
> Remember that the command word 'describe' means to 'give an account of or set out characteristics or features'. Ensure that you provide appropriate examples to support your response, related to vulnerable adults and the strategy for vulnerable adult care services during the pandemic.
> ▶ The context is a care home setting and the COVID-19 pandemic strategy for residents' care.
> ▶ Your answer needs to consider the impact of the pandemic on vulnerable adult residents.

Now write your answer in full.

....
....
....
....
....
....
....
....
....
....
....

Long-answer exam-style practice questions

1 Barry has severe epilepsy. He requires rescue medication in case he does not come out of a seizure and is receiving long-term treatment and medication for his epilepsy.

Explain the application of evidence-based practice (EBP) and how this could benefit Barry. Include relevant examples. (9 marks, plus 3 for QWC)

2 There are various sources of funding for the private healthcare sector and these have implications for access, quality and equity in healthcare.

Analyse the advantages and disadvantages associated with private sector funding and give specific examples. (9 marks, plus 3 for QWC)

A3 Health, safety and environmental regulations in the health and science sector

Recall activities

1 Match each hazard pictogram to its meaning. The first one has been done for you.

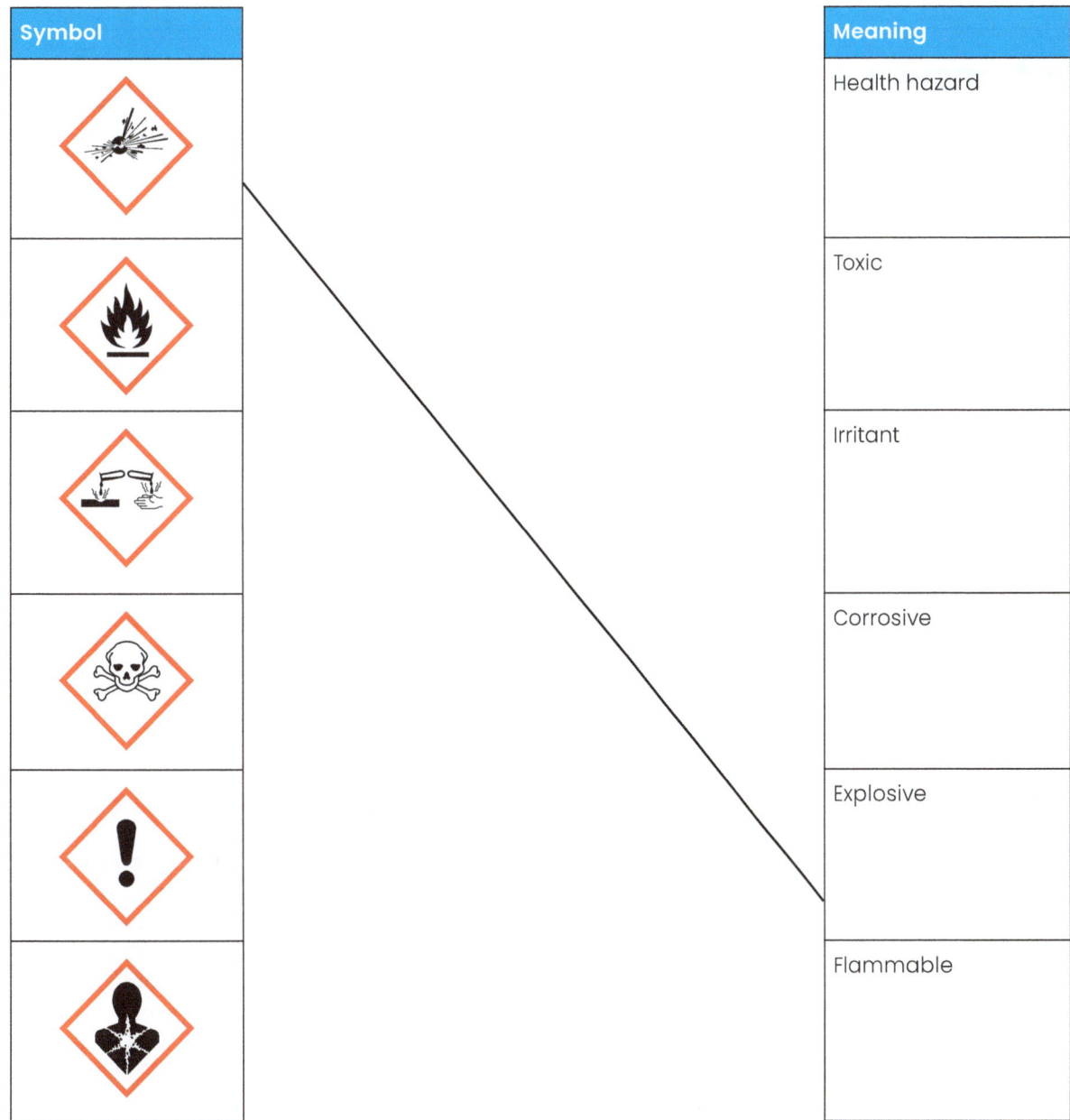

2 Read the statements below about COSHH regulations and tick to show whether they are true or false.

Statement	True	False
a COSHH applies to all substances that are hazardous to health, including chemicals, fumes, dust and biological agents		
b COSHH only applies to substances that are classified as toxic or hazardous by regulatory agencies		
c Employers are not required to monitor the health of employees who work with hazardous substances		
d Employers must provide appropriate PPE to employees who work with hazardous substances		

Short-answer exam-style practice questions

1 Define the term 'hazard'. (1 mark)

....

2 What does the acronym RIDDOR mean? (1 mark)

....

....

3 What may be classed as a reportable incident? (2 marks)

....

....

....

....

4 Identify the five steps of a risk assessment. (5 marks)

....

....

....

....

....

....

Tip

Each step in the risk assessment is worth 1 mark. Ensure that you understand the process and the necessary documentation that needs to be completed. Bullet points are acceptable.

A3 Health, safety and environmental regulations in the health and science sector

5 State **three** examples of who is responsible for the safety of everyone in the workplace, according to the Health and Safety at Work etc. Act (1974). (3 marks)

....

....

....

Long-answer exam-style practice question with scaffolding

1 Sarah has started a new role as a senior member of staff in a nursing home. She is aware that she needs to supervise the staff team to monitor and maintain health and safety regulations. Summarise how Sarah can ensure health and safety is promoted throughout the nursing home. (6 marks)

> **Sample answer**
>
> Health and safety at work is a critical consideration in healthcare settings to ensure the wellbeing of both employees and patients. The promotion of health and safety in the workplace involves various measures and practices aimed at preventing accidents, injuries and the spread of infections. All employees should receive comprehensive training on health and safety protocols. This includes training on the proper use of equipment, handling of hazardous materials, infection control practices and emergency procedures. Ongoing education ensures that employees stay informed about the latest safety guidelines.
>
> **Comment**
>
> This is the student's first paragraph. It is only a partial response and could be expanded upon. It could be more specific and concise in its explanations. This answer requires clarification as it is very generic and lacking in detail. Remember to consider such factors when constructing your own answers. This response could achieve 6 marks, but it needs to reference the scenario and give more specific examples.

Now write approximately four more lines to extend the answer by linking it specifically to the nursing home.

....

....

....

....

....

....

....

Long-answer exam-style practice questions

1. Graham works in a behavioural unit and encounters a confused and aggressive patient in a communal area. Explain how Graham might deal with this situation to avoid harm being caused to himself or others. (9 marks, plus 3 for QWC)

> **Plan your own answer**
> Make some brief notes on what your answer should include.
> ▶ Does your answer cover examples of Graham's possible response to the aggressive patient?
> ▶ Have you suggested specific actions Graham could take?
> ▶ Have you referred to teamwork to help with the situation?

Now write your answer in full.

A3 Health, safety and environmental regulations in the health and science sector

2   Stacey is on work experience on a hospital ward. Describe **three** relevant examples of health and safety legislation and regulations in the health and science area. (9 marks, plus 3 for QWC)

Plan your own answer
Write a rough draft of your answer to this question.
- Have you named and described three relevant examples of health and safety legislation and/or regulations?
- Have you linked the legislation/regulations to the question scenario?
- Look at the marks available for this question. Is there anything you could add to gain more marks?

....
....
....
....
....

Now write your answer in full.

....
....
....
....
....
....
....
....
....
....
....
....
....
....

A4 Health and safety regulations applicable in the healthcare sector

Recall activities

1. Complete the following statement regarding manual handling regulations. Use the words provided to fill in the gaps.

harm	insurance	protect	important
mandatory	healthcare	moving	

   It is .... to follow policy and guidance when .... equipment or other objects or positioning people. This is to .... the patients and .... professionals from .... This means that .... requirements should be met for .... purposes.

2. Define the term 'wellbeing'.

   ....
   ....
   ....

Short-answer exam-style practice questions

1. What must employers have by law to provide compensation to staff for injuries suffered in the workplace? (1 mark)

   ....
   ....
   ....

   Tip
   These are straightforward, low-mark answers and do not require in-depth analysis. They should only require a couple of sentences or a specific number of examples, for example, two examples for a 2-mark question.

2. State **two** purposes of workplace health and safety regulations in the healthcare sector. (2 marks)

   ....
   ....
   ....

A4 Health and safety regulations applicable in the healthcare sector

3 Why might employers provide an onsite automated external defibrillator (AED)? (3 marks)

....

....

....

....

Long-answer exam-style practice question with scaffolding

1 Samantha is a trained first aider working in a care service for young people on the autistic spectrum. One of the service users, Taj, has burnt his hand on a boiling kettle. When Samantha arrives, Taj is upset and says his hand really hurts.

Explain Samantha's general responsibilities as a trained first aider dealing with this situation, while following best practice. (6 marks)

> **Tip**
>
> Does your answer link to the scenario? Have you referred to 'best practice'? Have you explained at least two roles/responsibilities of Samantha?

Plan your own answer

- Six marks are allocated for a response, so ensure you have at least three distinct points in your answer. These points need to be well explained and refer to the scenario described.
- Think about the health and safety requirements Samantha needs to consider, as well as ethical concerns and administrative roles.
- Remember, Samantha needs to consider the responsibility of her own safety, too.

Use this space to make some notes:

....

....

....

....

Now write your answer in full.

....

....

....

....

....

....

Long-answer exam-style practice question

1 Tim has recently commenced work at a residential care home. All new staff must undertake relevant health and safety training and familiarise themselves with relevant policies, procedures and legislation. Why is the Care Act 2014 an essential part of this? (6 marks)

A5 Managing information and data within the health and science sector

Recall activities

1. List **eight** common methods used to collect data.

   1. ....
   2. ....
   3. ....
   4. ....
   5. ....
   6. ....
   7. ....
   8. ....

2. Create a mind map to identify how personal information is protected by data protection legislation, regulations and organisational policies.

   > **Hint**
   >
   > Can you name two pieces of legislation that protect personal information? Can you remember three ways organisational policies ensure compliance with legislation?

   How personal information is protected

Health T Level Exam Practice Workbook

Short-answer exam-style practice questions

1 a State **one** type of data that a healthcare practitioner could collect. (1 mark)

....

b Identify the **most** appropriate way to present data related to worldwide causes of death from disease. (2 marks)

....

....

....

2 Identify **two** ways that health apps support the healthcare sector. (2 marks)

....

....

3 List **three** advantages of using IT systems to record, store and retrieve information and data. (3 marks)

> **Hint**
>
> Remember that when you are asked to 'list', you do not have to write complete sentences. You can use bullet points, with no need for further explanation.
>
> Think about how IT systems have improved and streamlined data management processes.

....

....

....

4 Emma is a senior healthcare assistant whose care home has recently moved over to online systems. She can see the benefits but is also wary of the risks associated with the management of patient data.

Describe **four** potential risks associated with online systems. (4 marks)

> **Sample answer**
>
> Well, there are risks with online systems. The whole security thing is hackers getting in and messing stuff up. Then there's the system crashing, which happens all the time. Also, sometimes nobody knows what's going on and it's too complicated. Plus, people make mistakes using these systems, like putting in the wrong info or something.
>
> **Comment**
>
> A poor-quality response. It is informal, without a professional tone. The scenario is not appropriately referenced and claims are made without evidence, for example the system crashing all the time. This answer appears as though it has been based on negative perceptions of IT systems. You must ensure that your points are valid and evidenced in a professional manner. Always take time to consider tone and context.

A5 Managing information and data within the health and science sector

> **Plan your own answer**
> - What mark would you give the above answer? Why?
> - What improvements could you make?
> - Use the space here to make some notes.
>
> ....
> ....
> ....
> ....

Rewrite the sample answer to gain a higher mark – present the answer in three paragraphs.

....
....
....
....
....
....
....

Long-answer exam-style practice questions with scaffolding

1. A local GP surgery is planning to promote its smoking cessation programme – 'Time to Stop Smoking' – through social media channels. Discuss the ways in which social media could positively support the programme and what restrictions may limit this. (9 marks, plus 3 for QWC)

> **Plan your own answer**
> Your answer must relate to the scenario: patients at a GP surgery, stopping smoking and social media. Make notes on what you will cover in the full answer, using the following to help you:
> - Benefits of using social media to reach patients.
> - Negatives of social media, for example patient privacy concerns, whether all patients will be familiar with using social media.
> - A conclusion which weighs up the pros and cons of the use of social media for the smoking cessation programme.
>
> ....
> ....
> ....
> ....
> ....

Now write your answer in full.

....
....
....
....
....
....
....
....
....
....
....
....
....
....
....

2. It is common for large data sets to be collated for analysis within the healthcare sector. This includes tracking and monitoring patients' physiological data.

   Describe **three** different types of modern technology that are used to collect data and why they would be suitable. (6 marks)

> **Sample answer**
>
> Mobile apps offer user-friendly interfaces for capturing, organising and reporting data on the go. In healthcare, clinicians use mobile apps to record patient data, access electronic health records and report real-time updates.
>
> AI is used in analysing medical images such as X-rays, MRIs and CT scans.
>
> Cloud-based systems in healthcare involve the storage, management and processing of healthcare data on remote servers accessed via the internet. These systems offer many advantages, including improved accessibility, collaboration and scalability.
>
> **Comment**
>
> This is not a very strong answer, as it does not relate to the specific scenario. It is a generic answer and misses the point of the question, which is to identify specific technology and its uses. It may be worth up to 2 marks for the information given on the use of mobile apps and cloud-based systems, although the response regarding AI is very brief and lacking context.

A5 Managing information and data within the health and science sector

Plan your own answer
- Make sure that you include positive and negative examples.
- Think about misinformation and compromising patient confidentiality.

Positive examples	Negative examples

Now write your answer in full.

....
....
....
....
....
....
....
....
....
....

Long-answer exam-style practice questions

1 Freddie is a health practitioner who wants to gather quantitative data regarding outpatient procedures. He wants to know the impact of these on ensuring patient compliance prior to an outpatient procedure. Freddie is gathering three types of data:

  ▷ hard-copy patient questionnaires available on the ward
  ▷ patient emails
  ▷ direct interviews with healthcare practitioners.

Analyse the strengths and limitations of these sources in terms of providing accurate data.
(9 marks, plus 3 for QWC)

A5 Managing information and data within the health and science sector

2 Jamila is a support worker in a residential care home. She frequently needs to access a shared computer to update patient data. Jamila does not have full access to the system and more senior staff have different levels of access permissions. Explain how the care home could maintain confidentiality in this situation. (9 marks, plus 3 for QWC)

Tip

Use the mark scheme to mark your answer. Do you think it is a high-level answer? Why or why not? Can you think of anything extra to improve your answer?

A6 Managing personal information

Recall activities

1. Draw a line to match each data protection right to its corresponding meaning.

Data protection right
Right to be informed
Right of access
Right to rectification
Right to erasure
Right to restrict processing
Right to data portability
Right to object
Rights related to automated decision making, including profiling

Meaning
Can request the deletion of data
Can request data is transferred between organisations
There are controls about the automated collection and use of data
Must be allowed to see the data held
Can stop data from being used
Inaccurate information must be corrected
Can request data is not used
Must be told data is being collected

2. Complete this mind map to show reasons why personal information is collected in healthcare settings.

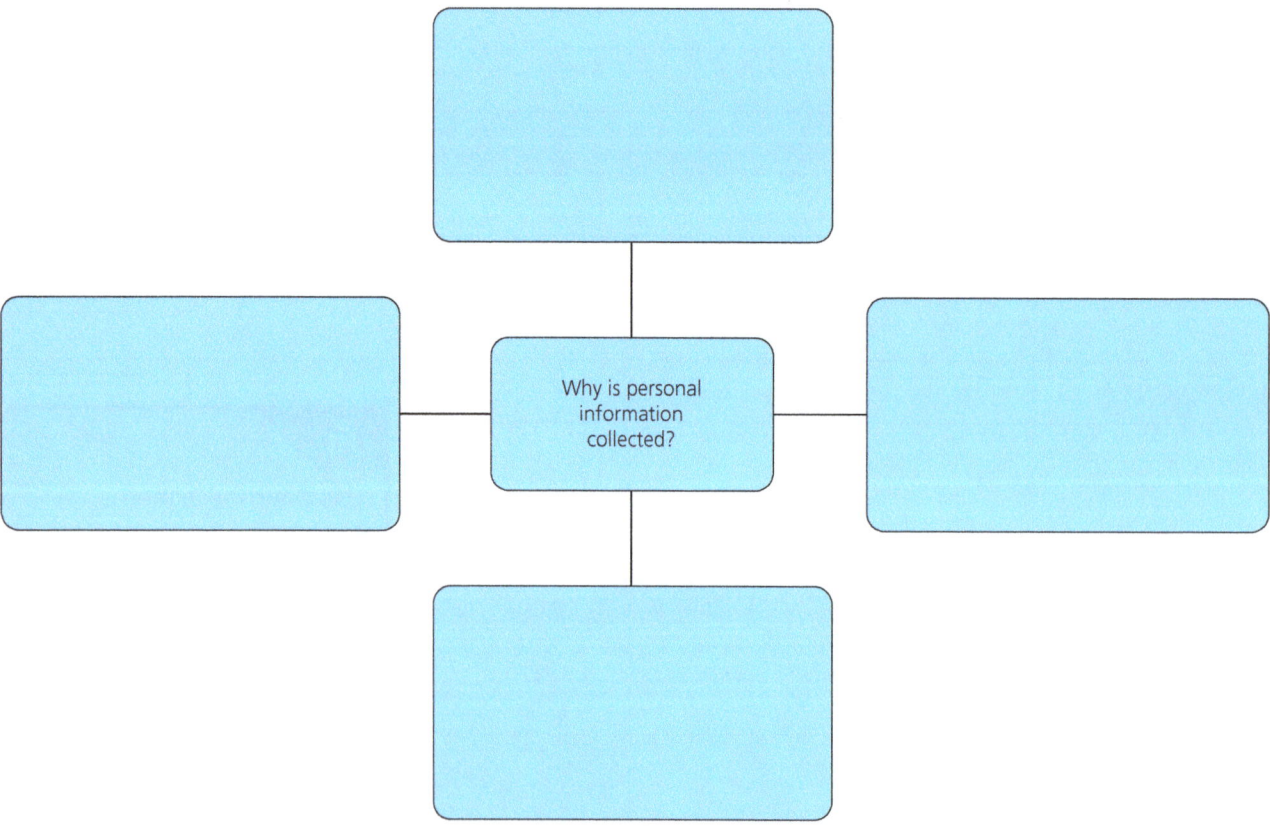

Short-answer exam-style practice questions

1 Why is it recommended to avoid using abbreviations when record keeping? (2 marks)

> **Sample answer**
> *Abbreviations are open to misinterpretation.*
>
> **Comment**
> This answer is very brief and would not gain full marks. The response could mention personal abbreviations, which would not be understood by anyone else. It could also suggest an agreed list of abbreviations that are clearly defined and used uniformly. Clarify that they can save time and be of use, provided everyone understands them. Alternatively, in some settings, no abbreviations should be used. Although this is only a 2-mark question, it still requires a clear, well-explained response.

Now write your own answer.

....

....

....

2 List **three** types of information required to obtain client history. (3 marks)

....

....

....

3 Describe **three** features of accurate records. (3 marks)

> **Tip**
> Read all questions carefully. The number of marks shown relates to the number of points of information expected. 'Describe' questions require you to give an account of or set out characteristics/features. To be awarded full marks you must describe three different features.

....

....

....

....

Health T Level Exam Practice Workbook

Long-answer exam-style practice question with scaffolding

1 Giovanni has just started a new role as a healthcare assistant in a hospital. He is attending his first shift handover and has been made aware of how important detail and accuracy is. Discuss the advantages of reporting systems for managing information in healthcare with regard to events, incidents and conditions. (6 marks)

> **Plan your own answer**
>
> ▶ Start by defining what is meant by reporting systems. You should include at least six points in your answer.
> ▶ Demonstrate that you have understood how each advantage is relevant in this situation.
>
> Use this space to make some notes.
>
> ....
> ....
> ....
> ....
> ....

Now write your own answer.

....
....
....
....
....
....
....
....
....
....
....
....

A6 Managing personal information

Long-answer exam-style practice questions

1 Kemi has complex needs and is extremely vulnerable. She has recently been moved from an emergency hospital admission to a new care provider. A large care file has been compiled detailing her needs, and the staff team are required to sign to say they have read Kemi's file and are aware of her needs. Evaluate the key reasons for keeping records and how this may contribute to Kemi's overall care. (9 marks, plus 3 for QWC)

> **Tip**
>
> Ensure that you understand the command verb and can apply your knowledge to satisfy the required assessment method. In this instance, you are required to evaluate, which means to review information and bring it together to make judgements and conclusions from available evidence. You must therefore apply your knowledge in a focused way, appropriate to the given scenario.

2 Simon is a vulnerable adult who has a learning disability. Simon can become distressed and confused, and display challenging behaviour during these times. While considering the need for confidentiality, assess when it may be necessary to share information on Simon with others and what needs to be considered when making these decisions. (9 marks, plus 3 for QWC)

A6 Managing personal information

3 Ibrahim works in a GP surgery and has responsibility for confidentiality and safeguarding of patient information. Analyse the responsibilities of employees and employers in relation to record keeping which Ibrahim needs to be aware of, and when it may it be necessary to escalate issues. (9 marks, plus 3 for QWC)

A7 Good scientific and clinical practice

Recall activities

1 Why is it important to follow standard operating procedures? Complete this spider diagram to show appropriate reasons.

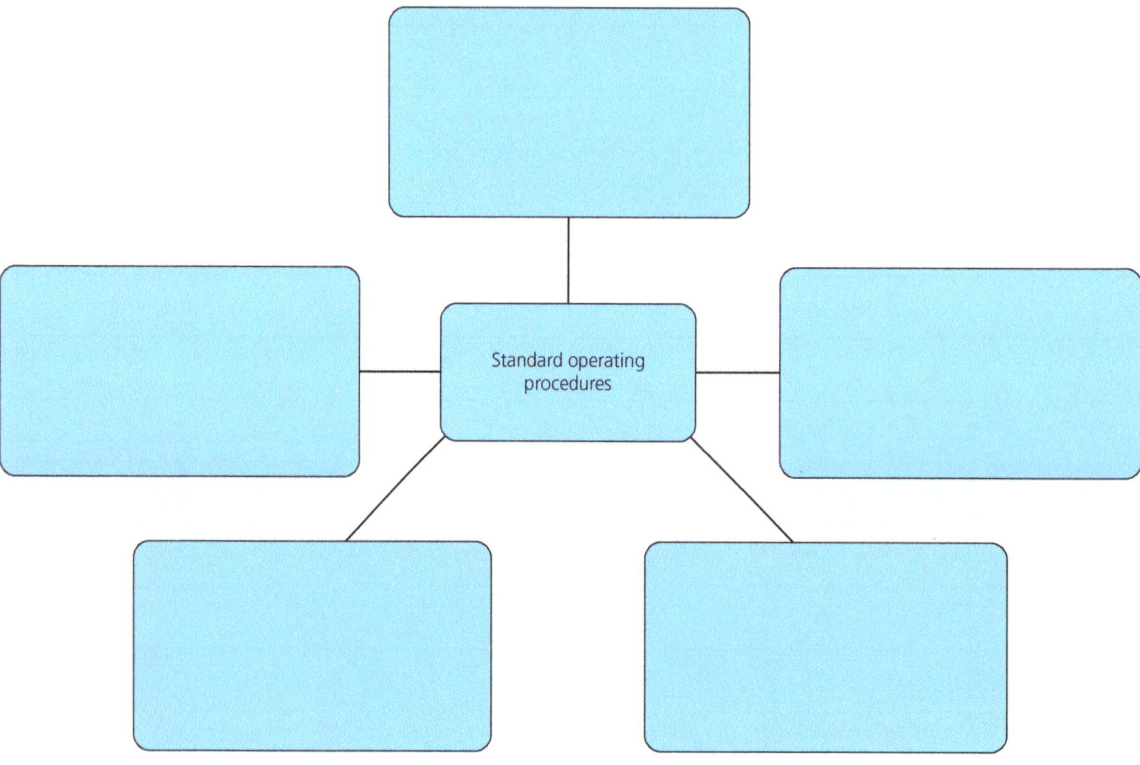

2 Which **two** of these are potential impacts of not maintaining, cleaning and servicing equipment effectively?

   a Increased risk of injury

   b Additional staff costs

   c Contamination or cross-contamination

   d Use of incorrect equipment

3 What is meant by an accurate measurement?

   ....
   ....
   ....

Short-answer exam-style practice questions

1. State **two** reasons why you may need to manage stock. (2 marks)

   ....

   ....

2. What is meant by the term 'standard operating procedure (SOP)'? (2 marks)

   ....

   ....

3. List **three** of the main principles of good practice in scientific and clinical settings. (3 marks).

   ....

   ....

   ....

4. A pathology laboratory maintains standardised protocols, including cleaning all equipment before and after use. Summarise **four** reasons why it is essential to clean equipment in this way. (4 marks)

   Hint

   Consider risks and dangers, especially in a laboratory environment. Think about both the impact on the equipment and the staff who may come into contact with it. How significant are the risks?

   ....

   ....

   ....

   ....

   ....

   ....

5. A nurse in a clinical environment comes across a BP monitor that is not correctly calibrated. How would they correctly respond to this? (4 marks)

   ....

   ....

   ....

   ....

   ....

   ....

Health T Level Exam Practice Workbook

Long-answer exam-style practice question with scaffolding

1   A health practitioner finds a broken blood pressure monitor. Outline why timely, scheduled maintenance is essential when considering the use of specialist equipment. (6 marks)

> **Plan your own answer**
> ▶ What is the impact of the broken monitor on the health practitioner?
> ▶ What are the risks associated with poorly maintained equipment?
> ▶ Make sure you construct a detailed answer, rather than just individual points. Consider performance and safety as well as compliance with organisational policy and procedures.

Now write your own answer.

Long-answer exam-style practice questions

1   A bottle of bleach is left in reach of adults with learning disabilities in a care setting. This could put service users at risk.

Analyse what may occur if safe, secure and effective storage mechanisms for dangerous products and materials are not in place. Provide appropriate examples and back this up with evidence. (9 marks, plus 3 for QWC)

A7 Good scientific and clinical practice

2. Jeremy is a healthcare assistant who is regularly monitoring a patient's temperature. Jeremy is obtaining wildly varying results.

   Evaluate the importance of correctly calibrated equipment when conducting physiological measurements in a healthcare setting.

   Your response should include:
   ▷ reasoned judgements
   ▷ conclusions about the impact of using correctly calibrated equipment. (6 marks)

A8 Providing person-centred care

Recall activities

1 Complete the table with definitions of the following terms:

Value	Definition
Empowerment	
Protection	
Prevention	
Proportionality	
Partnership	
Accountability	

2 List the NHS core values.

....
....
....
....
....
....
....

3 Draw lines to match the regulatory body acronym with the correct description.

Acronym
GDC
NMC
HCPC
CQC

Description
Organisation that regulates 15 health-related professional roles, including paramedics, physiotherapists, occupational therapists and speech and language therapists
Independent regulator that monitors, inspects and rates services and can take action if failings are found
Professional regulator of nurses and midwives in the UK and nursing associations in England
UK statutory independent regulator for dental care professionals

4 Read the statements about the responsibilities of each of the regulatory bodies and tick to show if they are true or false.

Acronym	Responsibility	True	False
CQC	Carries out inspections of hospitals and care homes to ensure standards are being met		
ICO	Independent Care Office for complaints and grievances		
Ofsted	Inspects and regulates social care services for children and young people		
HSE	Audits housing needs for young people		

Short-answer exam-style practice questions

1 State the purpose of the Mental Capacity Act (2005) plus Amendment (2019). (2 marks)

....

....

....

2 Explain the purpose of the Personalisation Agenda 2012. (2 marks).

....

....

....

3 Identify **two** potential barriers to communication. (2 marks)

....

....

....

4 State **four** of the six key principles of the Care Act 2014. (4 marks)

....

....

....

....

5 Identify **four** scenarios where the Liberty Protection Safeguards (LPS) would apply. (4 marks).

....

....

....

....

6 Define the following terms used regarding death and bereavement. (3 marks)

   a End-of-life care

   ....

   ....

   b Palliative care

   ....

   ....

   c Expected death

   ....

   ....

> **Tip**
>
> Consider those approaching the end of life. Has medication and treatment reached the point that it is no longer therapeutic? What actions might have an impact and what processes might make an individual in this situation more comfortable?

7 List **four** of the 6Cs in relation to person-centred care. (4 marks)

....

....

....

....

8 Identify **three** benefits of working within agreed professional boundaries. (3 marks)

....

....

....

A8 Providing person-centred care

Long-answer exam-style practice questions with scaffolding

1 Jim is a 25-year-old man with a learning disability. He struggles with communication and requires support with his personal hygiene. Evaluate how Jim's learning disability can influence his needs in terms of overall care. (9 marks, plus 3 for QWC)

> **Plan your own answer**
>
> It is essential to plan your response, incorporating key factors. You should include:
> - increased support requirements
> - behavioural factors
> - comprehension and communication.
>
> You should then evaluate your suggestions. Note that there is no 'correct' answer when evaluating, as long as you include relevant and reasoned arguments.
>
> Having a learning disability can significantly impact an individual's care needs, which can vary enormously, depending on the individual. Make notes below on some of these potential impacts.
>
> ....
> ....
> ....
> ....
>
> Now refer to the specific scenario and decide what Jim's needs are. Communication and hygiene are indicated, so person-centred plans need to be put into place for him. Write a paragraph based on what Jim's communication needs might be, their impact on his care and how support can help him.
>
> ....
> ....
> ....
> ....
>
> Additionally, identify Jim's potential hygiene needs. What support may be required and how does this impact on his overall care plan?
>
> ....
> ....
> ....
> ....

Now write your answer in full.

....
....
....
....
....
....
....
....
....
....
....
....
....
....
....
....
....
....

2 Explain how a healthcare practitioner could use the 6Cs to provide person-centred care to a service user who is on the autistic spectrum. (9 marks, plus 3 for QWC)

> **Sample answer**
>
> The answer below has been written by a student.
>
> Some of the 6Cs are compassion, competence, communication and caring.
>
> You need to use these to provide support for an individual. They should help you make that care specific to each patient. Person-centred care should help to improve health outcomes. Staff should build a better relationship. You must communicate appropriately and show that you really care. All staff must know how to apply these.

A8 Providing person-centred care

> **Comment**
> This sample answer is brief and lacking in factual content. It would only receive between 4 and 6 marks as it does not link to the given scenario, only mentions four of the 6Cs, and does not explain their use in any detail for the service user referred to in the scenario. For an 8-mark question, you must identify all of the factors and explain them, giving some examples of what they would mean in practice in this situation. Keep in mind the marks available when allocating time to write your answer. How many marks would you award this answer? Explain why.
>
> ....
> ....
> ....

Using the commentary and analysis above, now write your own answer to this question.

Long-answer exam-style practice questions

1. A healthcare practitioner is working with an individual who is in the late adulthood life stage. Describe what their typical care needs might be. (6 marks)

....
....
....
....
....
....
....
....

2. Describe how healthcare practitioners can support people with bereavement, considering a range of ways to communicate with families. (9 marks, plus 3 for QWC)

....
....
....
....
....
....
....
....
....
....
....
....
....
....

A8 Providing person-centred care

3 Explain how practitioners can promote independence and self-care for individuals. (9 marks, plus 3 for QWC)

....

....

....

....

....

....

....

....

....

....

....

....

....

....

4 Explain why it is important for healthcare assistants to maintain clearly defined boundaries with service users. (9 marks, plus 3 for QWC)

....

....

....

....

....

....

....

....

....

....

....

....

....

....

A9 Health and wellbeing

Recall activities

1. Create a mind map of signs and symptoms of pain, discomfort and deteriorating health and wellbeing in an individual. Include at least five signs and symptoms.

> **Hint**
> Remember there are verbal and non-verbal signs of pain as well as behavioural and physical signs.

> Signs and symptoms of pain, discomfort and deteriorating health and wellbeing

2. Use the clues to fill in the crossword regarding lifestyle choices.

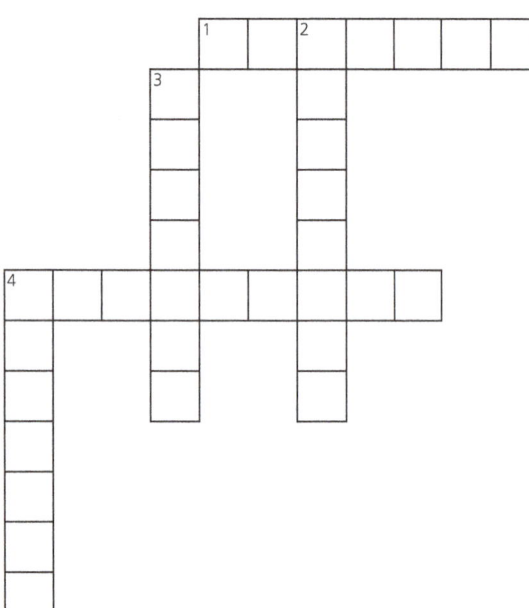

Across

1. Increases the risk of Type 2 diabetes, hypertension and heart disease (7)
4. Dependency on a particular substance (9)

Down

2. Lack of _____ can increase the risk of anxiety and depression (8)
3. One of the biggest causes of illness and death in the UK (7)
4. Long-term effects from this include damage to the heart, liver and pancreas (7)

Short-answer exam-style practice questions

1. List **two** ways in which health promotion can be used to support the prevention agenda and positive health and wellbeing. (2 marks)

   ....

   ....

2. State **three** methods involved in a holistic approach to healthcare. (3 marks)

   ....

   ....

   ....

> **Hint**
>
> The term 'holistic' means viewing something as a whole, rather than as a sum of its parts. It emphasises connections and the importance of understanding the entire system or entity to recognise its nature, function and behaviour.

3. State **three** lifestyle recommendations highlighted by the Making Every Contact Count (MECC) initiative. (3 marks)

   ....

   ....

   ....

4. State the BMI measures for the following categories: (4 marks)

   a Underweight ....

   b Normal ....

   c Overweight ....

   d Obese ....

5. List **three** ways signposting individuals to appropriate interventions or other services can support their health and wellbeing. (3 marks)

   ....

   ....

   ....

6. Describe the causes of **two** age-related diseases. (4 marks)

   ....

   ....

   ....

   ....

   ....

7 Identify the **two** main toxins present in cigarettes. (2 marks)

....

....

Long-answer exam-style practice questions with scaffolding

1 Teresa is a nurse looking after Andy who has had a stroke and requires support with daily tasks. Analyse how Teresa should work in a person-centred way to ensure adequate nutrition and care is provided to prevent deterioration in Andy's wellbeing. (9 marks, plus 3 for QWC)

> **Plan your own answer**
>
> Identify the command word required for this question. What specific features does it suggest you will need to include?
>
> ....
>
> ....
>
> ....
>
> ....
>
> Make a note of relevant examples of daily tasks before you start writing your answer. This should ensure that they are fresh in your mind.
>
> ....
>
> ....
>
> ....
>
> ....
>
> What are the key factors identified in the question?
>
> ....
>
> ....
>
> Now write some brief notes on how you might address these factors.
>
> ....
>
> ....
>
> ....
>
> ....
>
> Make sure that you review your answer and check that you have covered all points that are required.

Now write your answer in full.

....

(lined answer space)

2 Jamal is a heavy smoker and is overweight. His GP has advised him of lifestyle changes that could help him. On his way home, Jamal sees a government poster promoting public health and targeting both smoking and obesity. Evaluate the ways in which this poster may have an impact on Jamal. (9 marks, plus 3 for QWC)

> **Sample answer**
>
> This kind of advertising might make some people think about their issues. It could make people feel worse about themselves and that everyone was against them. Alternatively, it could help to reinforce a decision to make a positive change. It might prompt them to look for more help or contact a phone number or website.
>
> **Comment**
>
> This is a very brief response and is not directly linked to the scenario. Although it covers general themes, it is not a detailed answer, so would only achieve a low mark band, around 2–3 marks. The response needs to be linked directly to the scenario, emphasising the impact of the poster on Jamal. Including potential outcomes in terms of what it may prompt Jamal to do or not do, and the implications of any such actions, would enhance the answer.

Now write your own answer.

Long-answer exam-style practice questions

1. Lennon is a 4-year-old child within the age range of early childhood (3–8 years). Explain how care requirements for Lennon may have changed between infancy (0–3 years) and now.
(9 mark, plus 3 for QWC)

2. Peter is a 53-year-old man with bipolar disorder. Peter has a range of needs, requiring input from a variety of services. Analyse which methods would promote a holistic approach to Peter's care.
(9 marks, plus 3 for QWC)

3 Yusaf has been admitted to A&E after suffering from a fall. He is experiencing pain in his right hip and is not feeling well in himself at all. Yusaf's general health is deteriorating rapidly. Evaluate how to recognise signs and symptoms of pain and discomfort, while maintaining Yusaf's health and wellbeing. (9 marks, plus 3 for QWC)

A10 Infection prevention and control in health specific settings

Recall activities

1 Which of these is the minimum amount of time needed to effectively wash your hands?

   a   5–15 seconds ☐

   b   15–30 seconds ☐

   c   30–45 seconds ☐

   d   45 seconds–1 minute ☐

2 Define the term 'cross infection'.

   ....

   ....

   ....

3 Complete the mind map of good personal hygiene techniques in a healthcare environment.

[Good personal hygiene techniques]

Short-answer exam-style practice questions

1 Define the term 'antimicrobial resistance'. (2 marks)

   ....

   ....

2 Explain the purpose of disinfecting equipment in a clinical setting. (1 mark)

   ....

3. Tianna works on a busy hospital ward. She moves between several patients during her work and is aware of the need for infection control. What should Tianna always do before each patient contact and why? (2 marks)

....

....

4. State **four** safe sterilisation procedures used in clinical environments. (4 marks)

....

....

....

....

5. Norovirus is prevalent on a hospital ward. Omar is concerned for his safety and that of his patients. State **three** techniques Omar should use for infection control. (3 marks)

....

....

....

6. Describe **three** instances when an apron would need to be worn during personal patient care in a nursing home. (3 marks)

....

....

....

Long-answer exam-style practice questions with scaffolding

1. Evaluate the legal requirements of infection prevention and control. You should refer to appropriate legislation. (9 marks, plus 3 for QWC)

> **Sample answer**
>
> Infection prevention and control is an important aspect of healthcare and other industries where the risk of infectious diseases exists. Legal requirements are outlined in legislation to ensure the safety of individuals, prevent the spread of infections and maintain public health.
>
> For example, the Health and Safety at Work Act 1974. This legislation places a general duty on employers to ensure the health, safety and welfare of employees. It requires employers to conduct risk assessments, implement control measures to prevent infection and provide information, instruction, training and supervision regarding infection prevention.
>
> The Control of Substances Hazardous to Health (COSHH) Regulations 2002 focus on the control of substances that could be hazardous to health, including infectious agents. Employers are required to assess the risks, implement control measures and provide information and training to employees.

A10 Infection prevention and control in health specific settings

Additionally, RIDDOR (2013) includes specific provisions related to the reporting of work-related diseases, including those related to infection prevention and control. RIDDOR requires the reporting of specific infectious diseases. For example, if a healthcare worker is diagnosed with a notifiable disease due to occupational exposure (for example, a needlestick injury leading to bloodborne infection), it may be reportable.

Comment

This student's answer focuses on three pieces of relevant legislation. It could be expanded to give a more detailed response. The evaluation of legal requirements needs to include a range of relevant examples to achieve the higher level marks 9–12. You should understand infection prevention and control and this is the opportunity to demonstrate your knowledge base. This student's answer is quite general, so it may be possible to construct a more concise answer by focusing on the specific legal requirements and following this guidance. There is no evaluation, just descriptions.

Judgements and conclusions need to be made from available evidence. Evaluating something in detail involves a comprehensive examination and analysis of various aspects to gain a thorough understanding of its qualities, strengths, weaknesses and overall significance. You must clearly establish the criteria or standards against which you will assess the subject.

Now write your answer in full.

2 The NHS has a colour-coded scheme for hospital cleaning materials and equipment. Use this scheme to help you describe the essential rules for safe cleaning procedures in clinical environments. (6 marks)

Colour	Application
Red	Bathrooms, washrooms, showers, toilets, basins and bathroom floors
Blue	General areas including wards, departments, offices
Green	Catering department, ward kitchen areas and patient food service at ward level
Yellow	Isolation areas

Plan your own answer

▶ This is a 6-mark question, so you need to identify three rules and give a clear explanation of each to gain full marks.
▶ Consider what the colour-coded scheme tells you and how this can be used to respond to the question.
▶ Can you add other factors that are relevant, but not directly related to the colour-coding? Use of PPE, for example.
▶ Remember to make reference to appropriate legislation and regulations.

....
....
....
....
....

Now write your own answer.

....
....
....
....
....
....
....

A10 Infection prevention and control in health specific settings

Long-answer exam-style practice questions

1. Explain the scientific principles and processes behind cleaning, disinfecting, sterilisation and decontamination. (9 marks, plus 3 for QWC)

2. Discuss the impact of antimicrobial resistance, how this can influence infection control and how antimicrobial stewardship aims to prevent microbial resistance. (9 marks, plus 3 for QWC)

A11 Safeguarding

Recall activities

1. Draw lines to match the type of abuse or harm with the appropriate example.

Abuse/harm
Physical
Modern-day slavery
Sexual
Emotional
Coercion and control
Financial
Domestic

Example
Abuse that takes place in the home by a family member
Withholding/taking of money
Threats and intimidation
Female genital mutilation
Forcing someone to take part in or watch sexual activities
Exploitation of individuals for work using threats and violence
Gaslighting

2. Produce a mind map to identify how individuals and organisations can reduce the chances of abuse.

> **Hint**
> Think about policies and procedures. How can you improve their effectiveness? How can you focus the support for each individual?

Ways to reduce the risk of abuse

3. Identify the **six** key principles of safeguarding.

....

....

....

....

....

....

A11 Safeguarding

4 The table below states factors that contribute to abuse. Give a reason for each factor in the space below.

Factors that contribute to abuse	Reason
Age	
Health issues	
Lack of mental capacity	
History of abuse	
Social isolation	
Drug/Alcohol abuse	
Financial	

Short-answer exam-style practice questions

1 Define the term 'radicalisation'. (1 mark)

....

2 Define the term 'safeguarding'. (1 mark)

....

3 Explain why patient safety is important for clinical effectiveness. (4 marks)

....

....

....

....

....

> **Tip**
>
> For 2–4-mark questions, only include the information requested. You will not receive extra marks for further reasoning. Usually, 1 mark is awarded per factor identified.

4 Identify **two** signs of radicalisation. (2 marks)

....

....

....

....

5 Outline what is meant by a conflict of interest. (2 marks)

> **Sample answer**
>
> Where people do not agree on something important.
>
> **Comment**
>
> This is a 2-mark question, so does not require a long and detailed explanation but to receive the full marks you do need to give a brief explanation. This answer would only score 1 mark.

How could you improve this answer?

....

....

....

....

6 List **four** different types of abuse or harm. (4 marks)

....

....

....

....

....

....

Long-answer exam-style practice questions with scaffolding

1. Jules struggles to control his behaviour and can become increasingly frustrated. This is related to his limited verbal communication. Describe types of support for managing positive behaviour. (6 marks).

   Hint
   This is a 6-mark question, so you will need to identify three points, with an explanation of each. Ensure that these are relevant to Jules' communication needs and explain how they may help him to manage his behaviour. Remember to consider how Jules can be rewarded for positive progress.

2. Lucy is a vulnerable individual who lives in supported housing. Lucy struggles to make decisions and has been coerced and taken advantage of in the past. How could a social care practitioner use key safeguarding principles to protect Lucy? (9 marks, plus 3 for QWC)

   Sample answer
   Lucy's needs should be risk assessed, this helps to establish her needs and to identify types of care that would help. Lucy should be encouraged to contribute to decisions involving her care and support. Lucy should be supported by having information presented to her in an easy-to-understand format. An advocate would also help Lucy to make the right decisions for herself.

   Comment
   What mark would you give for this answer? Why?

   Suggest three ways this answer could be improved.

Now write your answer in full.

....
....
....
....
....
....
....
....
....

3 Describe the types and signs of abuse or harm and their impacts, that may be identified in individuals accessing healthcare services. (9 marks, plus 3 for QWC)

> **Hint**
>
> For a 12-mark question, you must ensure that your spelling, grammar and punctuation are accurate. Quality of written communication (QWC) is worth 3 marks, which is a quarter of the total marks available. Additionally, you should select three specific types of abuse or harm and describe each in detail, including what short- and long-term effects they could have on an individual.

....
....
....
....
....
....
....
....

....
....
....
....
....
....

A11 Safeguarding

Long-answer exam-style practice questions

1 Sonya is a healthcare assistant who has witnessed a patient being manhandled rather than being moved safely, following the correct procedure. Explain the relevant legislation, policies and procedures for supporting the safeguarding of individuals who need moving and handling. (9 marks, plus 3 for QWC)

> **Hint**
>
> Ensure that you refer to appropriate legislation. For example, how could the Mental Capacity Act (2005) help with the situation?

2 Sunita lives in a residential care home for older adults. Sunita is potentially at risk from abuse. Analyse what action should be taken if abuse is suspected or disclosed. (9 marks, plus 3 for QWC)

3 Discuss factors that may contribute to an individual being vulnerable to harm or abuse. (9 marks, plus 3 for QWC)

B1 Core science concepts

Recall activities

1. Fill in the gaps with the words below to explain the three principles of cell theory.

   | created | cells | basic | living | one | function |

   All .... things are made up of .... or more cells. Cells are the most .... unit of structure and .... in all living things. All cells are .... by pre-existing ....

2. Draw lines to complete the table to match micro-organisms with their average size and cell type.

Type of micro-organism
Bacterium
Fungus
Protist
Virus

Average size
20 nm – 350 nm
0.5 µm – 5 µm
5 µm – 50 µm
1 µm – 2 mm

Type of cell
Eukaryotic
N/A
Prokaryotic
Eukaryotic

3. What does DNA stand for?

   ....

4. What does RNA stand for?

   ....

5. What do ribosomes synthesise?

   ....

6. a What is the function of mitosis in nuclear division within cells?

   ....

   b How many nuclei does mitosis produce?

   ....

   c Are these nuclei named mother, daughter or sister nuclei?

   ....

   d How many chromosomes do they have?

   ....

7 Convert the following units of measurement:

   a 5 metres = ... millimetres

   b 100 millimetres = ... micrometres

   c 2 litres = ... millilitres

   d 6 millilitres = ... microlitres

   e 10 grams = ... milligrams

   f 100 milligrams = ... micrograms

8 Draw lines to match each classification system to the correct condition.

Classification system
Anatomical
Physiological
Topographical

Conditions classified
By bodily region or system
By organ or tissue
By function or effect

9 List the **five** key principles of homeostasis.

....

....

....

....

....

Short-answer exam-style practice questions

1 Define the term 'half-life'. (1 mark)

....

2 Which of these is the basic unit of proteins? (1 mark)

   a Monosaccharides ☐

   b Lipids ☐

   c Substrates ☐

   d Amino acids ☐

3 Below are four units of measurement. Which of these is **not** an SI unit? (1 mark)

   a Second ☐

   b Metre ☐

   c Litre ☐

   d Kilogram ☐

B1 Core science concepts

4 State **two** ways infectious diseases can spread globally among populations and communities. (2 marks)

> **Hint**
> This question is NOT looking for specific physical ways, such as sneezing or not washing hands. It is asking how diseases spread through various modes of transmission across populations.

....

....

5 Tallulah is a 58-year-old woman who is admitted to hospital with an elevated heart rate and blood pressure. What factors would a healthcare practitioner need to consider that could affect these physiological measurements? (4 marks)

> **Hint**
> Consider the impact of both genetics and lifestyle on health. How can people manage their health? Consider potential medical conditions, particularly those with a physical impact, as well as inherited disease.

....

....

....

....

....

6 Lindsay is a nurse and is preparing a patient for an MRI scan. Outline the procedures that Lindsay must follow before the patient is scanned. (4 marks)

> **Sample answer**
> When preparing for an MRI scan, patients must remove any jewellery and declare anything like a pacemaker that could cause problems.
>
> **Comment**
> This is a very brief and underdeveloped answer. It is written from the perspective of the patient, whereas the question asks about procedures from the perspective of Lindsay, the nurse. This answer would receive 1 mark for identifying one consideration.

Now write your own answer to this question.

....

....

....

....

....

Photocopying prohibited

Health T Level Exam Practice Workbook

7 Which type of pathogen is the causative agent for chlamydia? (1 mark)

   a Fungi ☐

   b Bacteria ☐

   c Parasite ☐

   d Virus ☐

8 In the image below, the actual measurement of the organelle is known to be 1.5 μm long.

You measure the image and find it to be 105 mm long. Calculate the magnification. (2 marks)

> **Tip**
>
> Remember to first convert the measurement from mm to μm by multiplying by 1000.

You can use the following equation to calculate magnification:

$$\text{magnification} = \frac{\text{size of image}}{\text{size of object}}$$

....

Long-answer exam-style practice questions with scaffolding

1 Jermaine is in a shared hospital room, recovering from abdominal surgery. Jermaine's roommate, Gavin, has a persistent cough and is sneezing frequently. Gavin coughs and sneezes without covering his mouth and also touches the bedrails, doorknobs and light switches without washing his hands. Analyse the different transmission methods that could lead to Gavin spreading pathogens to Jermaine. (9 marks, plus 3 for QWC)

> **Plan your own answer**
>
> Read the scenario and consider the command word, analyse, which means 'separate information into component parts'. Make logical, evidence-based connections between the components. Then make some notes on the key aspects of the scenario.
>
> ....
>
> ....
>
> ....
>
> ....

B1 Core science concepts

Next, identify three to four potential transmission methods.

....

....

....

....

Finally, make notes on how pathogens spread via the transmission methods you have identified.

....

....

....

....

Now use your notes to construct a full and well-written answer.

....

....

....

....

....

....

....

....

....

....

....

....

....

....

....

....

Photocopying prohibited

Long-answer exam-style practice questions

1. A pathogen is a micro-organism that causes illness or disease by damaging host tissues or producing toxins. Summarise the different ways in which pathogens may enter the body. (6 marks)

2. Homeostasis is the maintenance of an almost constant internal environment despite fluctuations in the external environment. Analyse how homeostasis contributes to maintaining a healthy body. (9 marks, plus 3 for QWC)

B1 Core science concepts

3 Describe the properties and functions of enzymes that are determined by their tertiary structure. (6 marks)

....

....

....

....

....

....

....

....

....

....

....

....

4 Throughout the COVID-19 pandemic, the government promoted initiatives such as 'hands/face/space'. Analyse how targeted awareness raising can help to prevent the spread of disease and disorder. (9 marks, plus 3 for QWC)

....

....

....

....

....

....

....

....

....

....

....

....

....

....

B2 Further science concepts in health

Recall activities

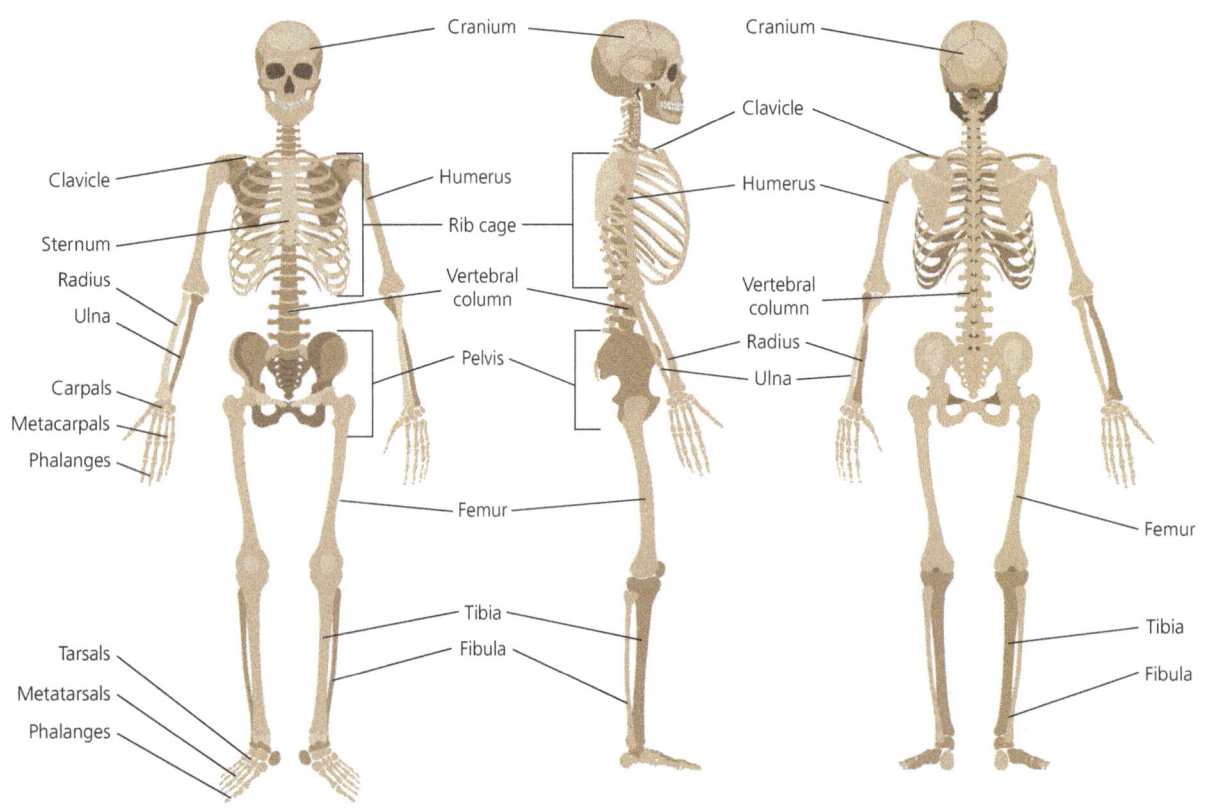

Figure 13.1 The full skeletal structure

1. Describe the following elements of the human skeleton.

Element	Description
Cranium	
Vertebrae	
Clavicle	
Sternum	

Element	Description
Rib cage	
Humerus	
Radius and ulna	
Pelvis	
Femur	
Tibia	
Fibula	

2 Construct a mind map to review your knowledge of rheumatoid arthritis.

Rheumatoid arthritis

3 List the **four** main symptoms of COPD (chronic obstructive pulmonary disease).

....

....

....

....

4 Label all the parts of the digestive system in the diagram below.

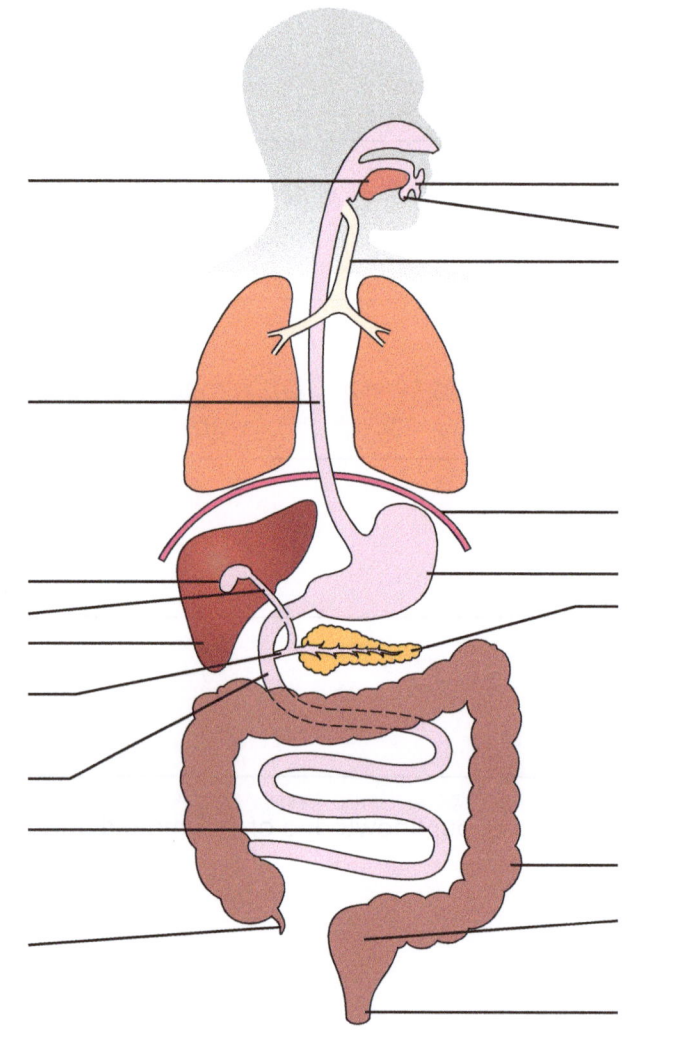

5 Match the missing words to this statement about the mechanism of blood glucose level control:

| insulin | concentration | other | glucagon | two | pancreas |

The .... produces .... hormones, insulin and ...., which are involved in the regulation of blood glucose .... The actions of .... and glucagon are antagonistic – they work in opposition to each ....

6 Define the following key terms:

   a Mutations

   ....

   b Genes

   ....

   c Dominant alleles

   ....

   d Recessive alleles

   ....

   e Sex-linked alleles

   ....

7 State the **four** elements of the composition of the blood:

   ....

   ....

   ....

8 Complete the table to explain the process of chemical digestion.

Enzyme	Location/source	Action
	Saliva (mouth)	Begins the digestion of starch into maltose
Pancreatic amylase	Pancreatic fluid	
Disaccharides		Convert disaccharides into their constituent monosaccharides
	Stomach and pancreatic fluid	Convert proteins into smaller fragments – peptides and eventually amino acids
Lipases		Break down lipids into fatty acids and glycerol

9   List the **five** main causes of Crohn's disease.

   ....
   ....
   ....
   ....
   ....

10 Label the diagram of the human respiratory system.

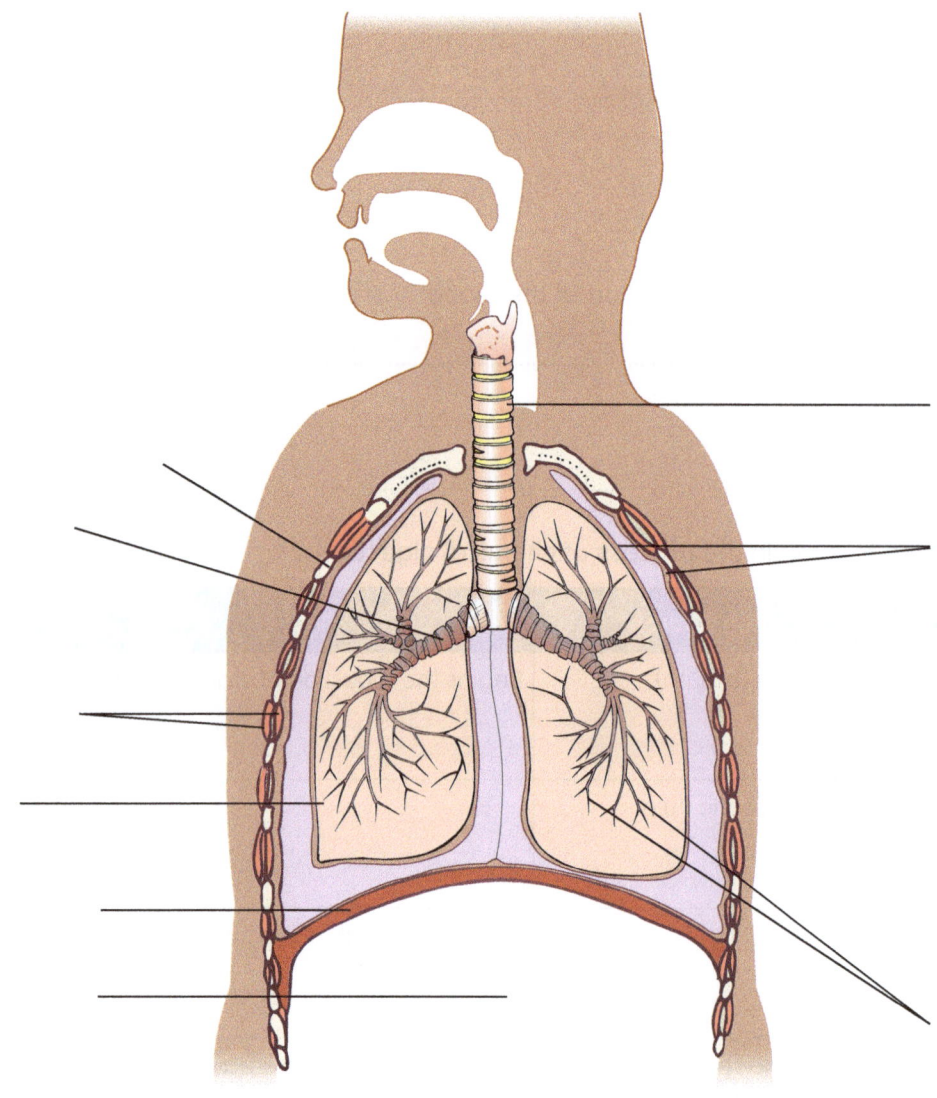

Short-answer exam-style practice questions

1   State **two** different treatment options for someone with muscular dystrophy. (2 marks)

   ....
   ....

B2 Further science concepts in health

2 Define the term 'diastole'. (1 mark)

3 Identify the **three** main types of diabetes. (3 marks)

4 Describe the **three** primary features of a motor neurone. (3 marks)

5 State **three** functions of the integumentary system. (3 marks)

6 Describe **four** common treatments for atopic eczema. (4 marks)

7 State the causes of endometriosis. (3 marks)

> **Hint**
>
> You do not need to provide a detailed explanation of what endometriosis is. You need to state three specific *causes* of endometriosis clearly and concisely. There is 1 mark for each cause, so even if you are uncertain of all three, you could pick up 1 or 2 marks.

8 Maddie is having symptoms of appendicitis and has been referred for a laparoscopy. Define the term 'laparoscopy'. (2 marks)

9 State the function of the male reproductive system and the **two** functions of the female reproductive system. (3 marks)

> **Sample answer**
> Men produce sperm and women produce eggs that help create a baby.
>
> **Comment**
> This answer is very simple and does not use appropriate terminology. Only one function of the female reproductive system is provided, so would receive only 1 mark. Consider what happens within the male reproductive system and try to expand upon this response. Can you add another function of the female system, related to the development of a foetus?
>
> ....
>
> ....

Now write your answer.

....

....

....

....

10 Describe the function of the following parts of the female reproductive system:

   a Fallopian tubes (1 mark)

   ....

   b Cervix (1 mark)

   ....

   c Vagina (3 marks)

   ....

   ....

   ....

11 Describe how semen is formed. (1 mark)

....

....

12 Describe the **three** distinct types of joint in the human body. (3 marks)

....

....

....

13 Dorothea is 65 years old. She presents to a GP with the following symptoms:
- chest pain (angina)
- shortness of breath
- generalised pain throughout the body
- feeling faint
- feeling sick (nausea)

Identify a likely diagnosis. (1 mark)

....

14 Explain the role of the following components of the endocrine system:

   a Pituitary (2 marks)

   ....

   ....

   b Ovaries (2 marks)

   ....

   ....

15 Describe the function of the endocrine glands. (1 mark)

....

16 Explain the difference between hyperglycaemia and hypoglycaemia. (2 marks)

....

....

17 Explain why a reflex action is classed as a survival response. (2 marks)

....

....

18 State the difference between benign and malignant tumours. (2 marks)

....

....

Long-answer exam-style practice questions with scaffolding

1. Graham is 43 and has recently developed Type 2 diabetes. Graham is overweight, single and currently unemployed. Discuss the impact diabetes may have on his body systems, as well as his mental and physical health. (9 marks, plus 3 for QWC)

> **Sample answer**
> Well, Graham being 43 and getting Type 2 diabetes is not great. This condition can mess with his body systems a lot. Blood sugars can be up or down. His heart might get weaker, his kidneys might struggle to filter stuff, his eyes could have vision problems, and his nerves might tingle. Graham's mental health might suffer, and he might feel tired all the time, struggle with weight loss or gain, and just not have as much energy as he used to.
>
> **Comment**
> This is a poor answer. It is very informal and does not use appropriate scientific language. The response is very generalised and does provides little insight or factual information. Although some of the statements are broadly correct such as, 'blood sugars can be up or down' and 'his eyes could have vision problems', the expectation at this level is for a much higher level answer. This response may achieve 2–3 marks for touching on a couple of relevant points, but needs further development. Think about the key points that should be included and the scientific terminology that needs to be used.

Now write your own answer.

B2 Further science concepts in health

2 Andy lives in a care home. He has had a fall and cut his forearm. Explain the functions of the relevant components of the integumentary system, in terms of how Andy's cut may begin to heal.
(9 marks, plus 3 for QWC)

> **Plan your own answer**
>
> The command term asks for an explanation of how the integumentary system works. What does 'explain' mean? Make a note below.
>
> ....
>
> What are the key factors that need to be considered in this scenario? Identify how you would address these.
>
> ....
>
> ....
>
> ....
>
> Make notes of terminology relevant to the integumentary system.
>
> ....
>
> ....
>
> ....

Now write your answer in full.

....

....

....

....

....

....

....

....

....

....

....

....

....

....

Photocopying prohibited

Long-answer exam-style practice questions

1. Meena is 38 years old. Meena's partner is infertile, so they are in the process of exploring IVF to conceive a child. Explain how the process of in-vitro fertilisation (IVF) could help them and what impact Meena's age may have on the outcome. (9 marks, plus 3 for QWC)

2. Allie is 67 years old and has developed rheumatoid arthritis. This particularly affects her right knee. Evaluate how common treatments could help to relieve Allie's symptoms. (9 marks, plus 3 for QWC)

B2 Further science concepts in health

3. Lucia is 16 years old and has been suffering with abdominal pains, fatigue and weight loss. She has recently been diagnosed with Crohn's disease. Lucia has experienced several upset stomachs recently and was hospitalised a month ago with severe food poisoning. There is a family history of multiple sclerosis and Lucia is concerned about this. Discuss the factors that are most likely to be related to the development of Crohn's disease in Lucia. (9 marks, plus 3 for QWC)

4. Mick is 56 years old and has had Parkinson's disease for five years. Although it can be a debilitating disease, he has been trying to develop ways to help him manage his condition. Analyse how Mick's Parkinson's could be managed to reduce the impact on his day-to-day life. (9 marks, plus 3 for QWC)

5   Rebecca is a 62-year-old patient with chronic kidney disease. Her GP has suggested that she needs to undergo dialysis and may require a kidney transplant in the future. Evaluate the potential impact on Rebecca of each of these treatments. (9 marks, plus 3 for QWC).

6   Helena is 18 years old and has muscular dystrophy. She displays symptoms such as muscle weakness and stiffness, difficulties in standing and walking, problems with swallowing and excessive tiredness. Discuss how common treatments could help to alleviate some of Helena's symptoms. (9 marks, plus 3 for QWC)

B2 Further science concepts in health

7 Explain the concept of sliding filament theory, in terms of proteins and muscle contraction. (6 marks)

....

8 Denise is admitted to hospital with an irregular heartbeat. She is concerned as to what this means and how it might affect her. Denise undergoes an exploratory procedure to investigate. Analyse the structure of the mammalian heart, in terms of how this could be described to Denise. (9 marks, plus 3 for QWC)

....

9 Saeed has indigestion and is feeling unwell. Evaluate how the human body breaks food down by physical and chemical digestion, and what may have caused Saeed's indigestion. (9 marks, plus 3 for QWC)

....
....
....
....
....
....
....
....
....
....
....
....
....

10 Tamsin has been diagnosed with an underactive thyroid by her GP. She is aware that this is part of the endocrine system related to her metabolism. Analyse the impact that having an underactive thyroid may have on Tamsin. (9 marks, plus 3 for QWC)

....
....
....
....
....
....
....
....
....
....
....
....
....

B2 Further science concepts in health

11. Morwenna is 61 years old and lives in a nursing home. Recently she has been displaying possible early symptoms of motor neurone disease. Discuss how these may manifest in Morwenna. (9 marks, plus 3 for QWC)

....
....
....
....
....
....
....
....
....
....
....
....
....
....

12. The renal system is responsible for several crucial functions in the human body. Analyse how the renal system regulates removal of waste products from the body. (9 marks, plus 3 for QWC)

....
....
....
....
....
....
....
....
....
....
....
....
....
....

13 Sarah is 14 years old and has recently visited her GP regarding the beginning of her menstrual cycle. Describe the growth and development of female reproductive characteristics which may be affecting Sarah. (6 marks)

....

14 Ellie is 24 years old and has a two-year-old child. Ellie is extremely concerned as she is about to undergo chemotherapy for invasive breast cancer. Ellie's mother also had breast cancer when Ellie was younger. Evaluate different courses of treatment that Ellie might receive. (9 marks, plus 3 for QWC)

....

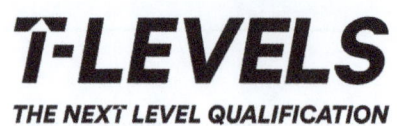

T-LEVELS
THE NEXT LEVEL QUALIFICATION

HEALTH: CORE
EXAM PRACTICE WORKBOOK

Develop the vital skills you need to achieve your best in the T Level exams with this accessible and engaging Exam Practice Workbook.

➡ Review and consolidate your knowledge, with varied recall activities for every topic including crosswords, mind maps and more

➡ Reinforce your understanding and boost your exam confidence with both short- and long-answer exam-style practice questions, to help you break down the question

➡ Improve your exam technique with guidance on how to plan and review your responses, plus exam hints and sample student answers

Also available:

9781036005115 Health T Level: Core Second Edition
9781398378940 My Revision Notes: Health T Level

'T-LEVELS' is a registered trade mark of the Department for Education.

'T Level' is a registered trade mark of the Institute for Apprenticeships and Technical Education.

The T Level Technical Qualification is a qualification approved and managed by the Institute for Apprenticeships and Technical Education.

 Visit us at **hachettelearning.com**

ISBN 978-1-0360-0698-3